Life Doesn't Have To Make You Sick

Life Doesn't Have To Make You Sick

Getting to the Root Cause...

Bryana C. Hillman

Writers Club Press
San Jose New York Lincoln Shanghai

Life Doesn't Have To Make You Sick
Getting to the Root Cause…

Writers Club Press
an imprint of iUniverse.com, Inc.

For information address:
iUniverse.com, Inc.
5220 S 16th, Ste. 200
Lincoln, NE 68512
www.iuniverse.com

No information in this book is intended to replace licensed or qualified medical attention. Always consult your physician before altering any course of treatment.

ISBN: 0-595-18494-4

Printed in the United States of America

Dedicated to women everywhere.

EPIGRAPH

The secret of health for both mind and body is not to mourn for the past, nor to worry about the future, but to live the present moment wisely and earnestly.

Buddha

CONTENTS

ACKNOWLEDGEMENTS

A special thank you goes to Doloris Casey for her editing and proofreading assistance, and also for her ceaseless support, input, and encouragement throughout the writing of this book.

I'd like to thank Julian Winston, editor of *Homeopathy Today* (a publication of the National Center for Homeopathy) for graciously giving me permission to include an article from the June 1998 issue.

Thanks also to Kathryn Petras, author of *The Premature Menopause Book*, for her positive support and professional tips.

INTRODUCTION

It's simply amazing to me how oblivious I have been concerning my own basic needs and self-undermining personality traits. I have spent most of my life doing what I've considered to be "the right thing", utilizing learned behavior and ideals acquired at an early age.

I felt compelled to write this book not only to help myself sort through the traffic jam of unwanted thoughts, emotions, and habits that sent me into a state of chronic anxiety and depression for close to a decade, but even more importantly, to possibly help others whose lives and health may be in a seemingly perpetual state of distress or imbalance.

Always wanting a logical and lasting resolution to any problem, combined with my own disappointment in the results I've received in the past through mainstream health care treatment which controls symptoms by suppression, I decided to embark on a personal journey toward healing myself using methods that would agree with my intelligence, intuition, and also my over-sensitivity to conventional medicine. Discovering and resolving the root cause of my ill health has come about slowly for me, through much self-education in the areas of natural and holistic health, and the mind/body connection itself.

Though particular non-traditional health therapies have helped me immensely, I don't suppose to imply that what works for me will work for you. I also don't believe that any healing medicine will indeed heal in totality without one's active participation in addressing and resolving the root cause that created the undesirable symptoms of dis-ease in the first place. Instead, I offer up my own layperson's story and insights: what I've learned and discovered through my own personal experience and suffering and the experience and suffering of others.

Whatever ails or troubles you, don't give up and don't give in. Have faith in yourself and a higher power, and realize that the ability is *within you* to create health and happiness for yourself. Remember life doesn't have to make you sick.

I

OUR HEALTH

SOME OF MY OWN HEALTH EXPERIENCE

There is nothing the body suffers that the soul may not profit by.
George Meredith

I grew up in Southern California, my family belonging to one of the largest health care providers operating in the West. The last of five children, I was the sickly one, the runt of the litter you might say. Between near-fatal toxoplasmosis, mumps, scarlet fever, chronic tonsillitis, long-term "mystery" viral conditions, frequent kneecap dislocations (genetic perhaps), a broken jaw (the result of a bicycle accident), and vision problems, I spent quite a lot of time in doctors' offices as a child. I don't remember deriving much benefit from these office visits, with the exception of the optometrist, though I probably avoided some possibility of secondary infections considering all of the antibiotics I was prescribed.

By the time I was in my mid-twenties I convinced my then family doctor that I needed my tonsils removed, as I was taking broad-range antibiotics six months of the year and pretty tired of the whole tonsillitis business by then. (I still had my tonsils in my twenties because it wasn't the medical trend to remove tonsils in the absence of chronic strep infections when I was growing up, at least not in the medical community I lived in.)

Unfortunately the ear, nose, and throat specialist that I was referred to for the tonsillectomy was, in my opinion, a morally depraved man who insisted on an unnecessary and unethical breast examination in front of

3

floor to ceiling undraped windows, which resulted in his announcement to me in a disappointed tone that I was underdeveloped. Upon lengthy and aggressive examination of my tonsils with a tongue depressor, he then patronizingly said, "Oh, you're a gagger". I shuddered off the thought of why he would care.

Like many women, I'm sure, that was simply one of several negative experiences with physicians of patronizing and/or perverse character that I have endured as a female patient. I won't recount some of the OB/GYN experiences I have also been subjected to. They are best left to the imagination.

I've included this one incident because I feel it is important for women to know that any morally or professionally questionable behavior that any medical professional confronts you with or tells you is "standard procedure" is not to be accepted or tolerated under any circumstances. Report unprofessional behavior to the medical authority that presides over the physician, and tell your friends and family, so others won't be needlessly subjected to a similar experience. I believe that oftentimes we put too much unquestioning trust in medical professionals and needlessly subject ourselves to unpleasant experiences because of that trust.

I also believe, however, that most people, no matter what profession they are in, are basically good and competent people. It's that small percentage of those who aren't that we need to guard ourselves against and expose if necessary.

At the age of 30, shortly after discontinuing long-term use of birth control pills, I developed chronic fatigue syndrome (caused by the Epstein-Barr virus, according to blood tests), chronic pelvic infections, ovarian cysts, and chronic headaches and migraines. When my family doctor told me that there was no available treatment for the virus, and when the prescribed antibiotics for the pelvic infections did nothing to stop their recurrence, and painkillers didn't resolve the migraines, I decided it was time to try something different, to make some sort of effort to heal myself.

I drove by a small shopping center containing a vitamin store every day on my way home from work. One day I just decided to stop and browse through the store before going home. I bought a book called: "Prescription for Nutritional Healing" by James F. Balch and Phyllis A. Balch, took it home and read it thoroughly. The next day I purchased all the essential nutritional supplements listed in the book for my particular health problems. By the eighth week of vitamin therapy, the symptoms I'd had for over a year disappeared completely. I was thrilled not only with the natural treatment modality, but also that for the first time in my life I took control of my health and met with successful results!

Over a year later, I found myself going through a tremendous amount of personal stress, involving both my marriage and work environment, and I had no support system at that time to help me ride out the "rough". I became pregnant (despite the fact that I had resumed regular use of birth control pills five months earlier) at a time when I was seriously considering dissolution of my marriage. The pregnancy gave me a positive event to look forward to, but certainly not under the best of circumstances.

As it turned out, I had a blighted ovum, and miscarried the pregnancy "remains" several months later, prompting an emergency D & C. Upon waking from the D & C anesthesia, I knew something was terribly wrong with me. I couldn't think clearly, my heart raced and palpitated, every nerve and muscle in my body was tensed, and my blood pressure was jumping from 230/120 to 80/50. Convinced that the blood pressure monitor had to be malfunctioning, the nurse proceeded to disconnect it and wheel it away, without ever checking my blood pressure again.

After being released from this day surgery and going home, my symptoms got progressively worse. I was admitted to the hospital a few days later for 24 hours of intravenous antibiotics because of infection, and was then again released to go home feeling even worse than before. I left my highly stressful job within three months, and sought help from my family physician, totally unaware of what was wrong, but guessing it might be some sort of hormonal imbalance. Baffled by the array of symptoms, he sent me to an OB/GYN who merely did a pap smear and announced its normal results. No hormone levels were measured because in his opinion I was too young to be having any hormone problems. I was then referred to an endocrinologist, who tested me for Diabetes and Graves Disease, with negative result, and simply noted on a sheet of paper in my file that I was hyperventilating at the time of the examination. He in turn referred me to an ear, nose, and throat specialist because of my lack of balance while walking. The ENT didn't speak at all during his examination; instead he handed me a prescription for thirty Valium without explanation, and referred me to a neurologist. The neurologist, also a non-communicator, did a series of tests that produced negative results, but went ahead and prescribed a succession of medications for me anyway, one of which caused me to hallucinate. (I immediately threw that particular prescription in the toilet and flushed thoroughly.)

None of these doctors diagnosed me, yet almost all of them wrote prescriptions for drugs which only served to exasperate some of my symptoms. After ten months of sleeping a maximum of four hours per week, being unable to eat without pain, bloating and severe nausea, experiencing rampant heart palpitations, hot flushes, chronic pelvic inflammation, migraines, an inability to concentrate, and the unbearable feeling of wanting only to scream and run, I was so miserable, confused and depressed, I reached a point where I didn't think I cared if I lived or not. Don't get me wrong, I was by no means suicidal in thought, simply desperate for an answer and resolution to the situation. It was the first time in my life (so many times I think desperation precedes the first time for people) that I talked to God. I said to God: (with only a weak sliver of hope still in me that there was indeed a God and that this supreme, benevolent, intelligent force might actually hear me and take action) "God, I can't stand this any longer. Please give me something to look forward to." Please keep in mind that during this ten month period after the D & C, I was home alone all day every weekday and for the most part, ignored evenings and weekends by my husband and preteen daughter because, I assume, of their inability to relate to me in the overall state of health I was in. Throughout this time I felt very alone and isolated.

Coincidence perhaps, but 3 days after my "talk" with God, I discovered I was pregnant again. Within the next 3 months my symptoms got about 80% better, and I delivered a wonderful, healthy baby girl 6 months after that. I enjoyed being a new mother again after 11 years, and loved taking care of this new little person in my life.

When the baby was about 18 months old, and my thirteen-year-old daughter came back from a summer trip spent back east with her best friend, I seemingly overnight went into the same terrible state of health I had been in before the pregnancy. With a toddler to take care of, I knew I could not allow this unbearable condition to take over my life again. I had to find out what was wrong and determine a course of action.

I went to a neighborhood urgent-care clinic and saw a female internal medicine physician who ran some tests which again all proved negative. But after listening to my description of the physical, mental, and emotional symptoms I was experiencing, she told me that I was probably having panic attacks. (Chronic panic, I found out later, was the actual state I was in.) I knew nothing at all about anxiety or panic, and hadn't ever known anyone who had panic attacks, so was clueless as to what I could do about the problem. I was, however, thrilled to actually have some kind of diagnosis after being in the dark for so long. The physician gave me a prescription for Atarax, an anti-anxiety drug, and told me to come back in a few months. The Atarax worked beautifully for many of my symptoms, until I got my next period. From that point on, it did absolutely nothing. At this point in time, I still felt that hormones might be playing some sort of role in all of this.

Desperate again (but this time armed with a diagnosis), I went to the same vitamin store I had gone to before, and bought appropriate nutritional and herbal supplements for anxiety. Unfortunately, they didn't improve my symptoms.

After several more months had passed, I happened to be in the vitamin store again and noticed a sheet of paper pinned to the wall behind the counter listing homeopathic physicians in the city. I had been to a homeopath a couple of years earlier at the recommendation of a co-worker, but found that the numerous remedies he prescribed were ineffective. One name on this list caught my eye however. In parenthesis next to the name was written: "classical homeopathy". I didn't know there was more than one method of prescribing homeopathic treatment, and I was more than a little interested. I jotted the number down and called the next day to schedule an appointment. The appointment consisted of a ninety-minute interview. I told the homeopath (also a licensed D.O.) about all of my symptoms, and handed him a blood work report along with the current medical history form I had filled out in the waiting room. I answered numerous questions about my symptoms, food and temperature preferences, fears, cravings, recurring dreams, likes and dislikes, family relationships, etc. This doctor prescribed one "constitutional" remedy for me in liquid form, which I began to take once a day. He told me that I might have an exacerbation of symptoms before I saw some improvement, which did indeed happen, but I gradually improved and realized that the remedy was working on mental and emotional levels that nothing else ever had. Slowly I became aware that my state of ill health was not only a matter of hormonal imbalance (a factor that I personally uncovered) but the result of a continual buildup of negative emotions and circumstances over the years. I experienced a sort of inner awakening throughout the next year and a half. I came to realize that the people and environments I had made the central focus of my life had been draining me physically, mentally, and emotionally over many years. As a result, my body really had no choice but to give me a wake-up call that would make me take notice.

I had stayed in personal and work relationships for years that were very detrimental to my health and well being, and had, in essence, suppressed thirty years of negative emotions and events. Though no medical treatment can resolve relationship problems, the proper constitutional homeopathic remedy and appropriate Bach Flower Essences not only brought me back to physical health, but also brought me to a state of mental and emotional awareness that allowed me to see that I needed to make some changes in my life to avoid chronic illness. My own added "prescription" of natural (non-prescription) progesterone cream in addition to the constitutional remedy and flower essences completed the healing picture for me, alleviating the physical and mental/emotional symptoms of premature menopause which had become very pronounced in me by the age of 35.

Reading this now, it's obvious to me what happened and why. But I believe that like many other people overwhelmed with a continual flow of negative circumstances over a long period of time, I at the time, couldn't see the forest for the trees.

I have since suggested classical homeopathy and Bach Flower Therapy to several other people I know with chronic health conditions as alternative/complementary treatment options. The main reason I am disclosing some of my own personal health experiences here, is to impress upon everyone (especially women who many times are not taken seriously or treated with the same respect as men by the medical community) the importance of exploring all available options when it comes to individual health care. Everyone is different, each of us unique. Since one method of medical treatment may work for one person but not another, we must take it upon ourselves to explore all of our options. Nutritional and herbal therapy, homeopathy, oriental medicine and acupuncture are only a few of the valuable and proven "alternative" or complementary treatment options available. I can't overstate the importance of *self-education* in matters of such importance as health care. Getting to the *root cause* of any problem and addressing or treating *it* is key. It has been my experience that suppressing symptoms only serves to compound or transform them. And, taking an active role in our individual health care cannot be overstated.

I would be thrilled if I lived to see the day where affordable integrated health care (which provided Americans with medical insurance that covered both conventional *and* non-conventional treatment options) became available to everyone in this country.

COMMON SENSE AND DEDUCTION IN HEALTH MATTERS

One often learns more from ten days of agony than from ten years of contentment.
Merle Shain

A lot can be said for using common sense as a strategy for creating and maintaining a state of good health. Getting enough sleep, eating natural as opposed to processed food, getting some exercise, etc., are just a few of the common sense methods used by most of us. Equally important, however, is the ability to deduce what may have caused a temporary or chronic state of ill health.

I used to get viruses quite often on weekends and holidays. I realized through simple deduction, that I became ill at those times because I was overtired, and I either consciously or subconsciously felt that weekends and holidays were the only time I was "allowed" to get sick while working a full-time job. When my work or home environment became especially stressful, I got migraines. Pelvic and bladder infections dominated when I was involved in a stressful relationship with a man. Feeling I was trapped in a negative situation or relationship, with no apparent available options out, gave rise to anxiety and depression.

I have learned over the past few years (with the help of constant journal writing) what events, circumstances, habits, attitudes, or even foods trigger illness or mental/emotional turmoil in me. Everyone can learn the same about themselves.

If you get a splitting headache every time you eat fajitas at your favorite local restaurant, it is apparent that you are sensitive to something in the fajita. If you become anxious or nauseated whenever you're in the company of a particular person you should avoid being with that person as much as possible. If you hate your job, ask yourself why, and then look hard for a different one while you're still employed. (If you don't determine why your current job is causing you excess stress, you may end up in the same situation at your next place of employment!) If you're depressed because you feel lonely, get involved in activities that provide you with an opportunity to meet people with similar interests and a positive outlook on life.

Stress is a major factor in the case of illness and disease. Writing in a journal every day (I simply use a spiral bound 3-subject notebook, nothing fancy!) is a practical tool that can be used to uncover patterns and determine the circumstances or events that precede your symptomatic conditions. Using a diary would likewise work, but I find that I have more to say about the average day than would fit on those little pages! When you write in a journal every day, you enable yourself to go back through the pages of time and see specific instances or situations that triggered a negative response in you.

If you have a chronic condition, or even if you just seem to spend more time in medical offices than you care to, take the time to review *all* aspects of your life. Thoughtful review utilizing common sense and your own powers of deduction can usually provide you with the answers you need to prevent many states of ill health from occurring or recurring. I find it equally important to take an honest look at one's own self-undermining personality traits. Doing this can enable us to understand and overcome the cause and effect of negative and/or self-defeating mindsets and emotions on the physical body.

"ALTERNATIVE" HEALTH AND TREATMENT OPTIONS

Perhaps in time the so-called Dark Ages will be thought of as
including our own.
G.C. Lichtenburg

The patenting of natural substances, as they are originally found in nature, is not allowed by law. As a result, the molecular alteration and synthetic reproduction of natural substances ensued and through the power of the patent, became the profitable method of producing medicine. Because of the advances in the science of medicine and human biology, many lives have been spared a premature or painful death, many diseases centuries old have been all but wiped out globally. Unfortunately, the use of molecularly altered and synthetically reproduced substances found in nature does not occur without the risk of negative side effects. Many existing diseases or ailments may be symptom-controlled with orthodox drugs, but with the overwhelming risk of adding on new symptoms and/or medical conditions which will require additional treatment. Medical science is an ongoing experiment in relieving human pain and suffering, in the preservation of health, and also in the quest for youthfulness and longevity.

There's a growing population of people in this country turning away from conventional medicine to natural non-invasive health care treatments and therapies. Tired of being treated only as mechanical organisms, fearful of physically and emotionally painful and invasive medical procedures, tired of and sickened by the often dangerous side effects of the allopathic medicines used today, people have developed a renewed interest in classical homeopathy, herbal medicine, acupuncture, nutritional therapy, oriental medicine, and a whole myriad of available health care treatment options that have been overshadowed and berated by our current "conventional" medical system for many decades.

The following condensed article entitled: "Violence, Medicine, and the Soul", from the June 1998 issue of Homeopathy Today (a monthly newsletter published by the National Center for Homeopathy in Alexandria, VA), reflects the current attitude of many Americans today:

"What do doctors have to do with souls? We are concerned only with bodies and ailments."

Doubtless some such querulous remark will be made, in sotto voice, by more than one of my readers, on glancing at the title of this paper.

The retort in kind, Yankee fashion, might be: "What has a plumber to do with the tenant of a house in which he is making some badly needed and rather expensive repairs? Who engaged the plumber to do the job? Who watched him rip up his walls and floors, fumble around in dark passages, cut out and replace pieces of damaged piping, clean out filth from obstructed traps and flush them, repair leaky faucets, etc., all the while wondering how much his bill will be and whether his bank account will stand it?"

The general drift of the people away from the medical profession is great and very rapid. Surveying the field covered by all the "no-drug," non-medical, anti-medical, religious and sectarian bodies and cults, and by the various newspapers and periodicals devoting more or less space to the subjects of health, hygiene and physical culture, it has been estimated that there are now more than thirty million people in the United States who have abandoned the medical profession within the last twenty-five or thirty years. That is something to think about.

Within the medical profession itself there are large numbers of physicians who not only resent and oppose the dominance of the little cliques of political schemers who rule their organizations, but sense with alarm the dangers to the true healing art inherent in this vast aggregation of capital invested in huge "medical centers", hospitals, clinics, "research" laboratories, institutes and foundations. They perceive more or less clearly that such institutions tend toward that pernicious state of centralization, standardization and fossilization which is the greatest obstacle to real scientific progress, and is destructive of personal liberty. With these opposing forces organized medicine is waging a constant warfare and must continue to do so. Victory for either is "in the lap of the gods," but who can doubt that in the end American ideals will prevail?

Dominated by a coldly materialistic underlying philosophy which does not give a thought to the soul of man, and using the analytical methods of modern physical science, medicine today dismembers, dissects and disintegrates the human body into its material elements to such an extent that all sense of human form and individuality is lost. Chemists rob the body of its form and reduce it to a few pathetic little piles of earthy substances—"earth to earth and ashes to ashes." They may also secure a jar or two of invisible gases, but the life principle, the man himself, the form and soul of him, eludes them.

Histologists tear and tease organic tissue to tatters, and under the microscope scan its cells and fibers, but never succeed in bringing their formative principle into view nor in gaining any knowledge of its nature. Lacking imagination, they see connective tissue but are blind to connective principle. They clutch at the shadow but do not find or see the substance.

The habitual mode of approach to man himself is so cold-blooded, so precipitate, so essentially rough and brutal, that he is frightened away. He may submit his body for examination, but his soul retires into its citadel and refuses to reveal its secrets.

A physical examination nowadays is a fearsome thing. No wonder the average mortal dreads it. It is so complex and technical that no one man can perform it. To do it to the complete satisfaction of the directors of Gotham Diagnostic Institutes or the Life Elongation Societies requires the use of a large building, an appalling array of equipment, and a crowd of nurses, attendants, "experts" and technicians, none of whom, you may be sure, works for the love of it. Like the witty Irishman in the trench who was asked by a simpleton what he was diggin' for, most of them might truthfully reply as he did, "Diggin' for dollars, sor."

From the outsiders' standpoint, or even for some who are "on the inside," there is a ludicrous side to this, as there is to everything which is carried to extremes. Much of it is totally unnecessary for the real physician, mere "grandstand play." Staged for the purpose of drawing the crowd and increasing the receipts at the box office. Observe how, as they hustle him through the various departments, or "side-shows" of this diagnostic circus, they undress a man, inspect him, auscultate, palpate and percuss him; lay hold of and throw him down bodily; stick their fingers, probes and specula into his orifices and passages; light up his cavities and interiors and peer into them; "flash a dark lantern" on him like the old-time highwayman, holding him up before a fluoroscope to watch his private internal actions; steal samples of his blood, his secretions and his excretions; ram a rubber tube down his throat and despoil his stomach of a tantalizing "test meal," etc.; all without the slightest apparent regard for his dignity, his feelings or his pocketbook.

In short they treat him much as the inspectors of an African diamond mine treat a native laborer before he is permitted to leave the stockade at the end of his contract period. He may or may not have picked up and attempted to secret a precious stone somewhere on or in his naked person. He is considered guilty until he is proven innocent. Some of the things done to him must be left to the imagination. Suffice to say that when the inspector gets through with him, the poor wretch knows something about a "thorough examination." He may even be a candidate for the hospital.

Funny, isn't it, when you look at it that way? Especially when you recall (if you are a follower of Hahnemann) that many of these showy, elaborate, painstaking and frequently painsgiving procedures yield nothing that is of value or use in selecting the curative remedy.

The objection here, of course, is not so much to the examination itself as to the manner and spirit in which it was done, to the use made of its findings, and to the ignoring of subjective phenomena—in a word, of the man himself.

Physicians and surgeons have so long looked upon man as a machine, a physical, chemical and mechanical laboratory, that many of them have become callous. They have lost sight of the soul of man, of the individual ego, of Life and its processes, and hence have gone far astray and failed to find the key to the problem of real healing. Whether they are aware of it or not, they are denied access to the inmost citadel of life, which they try to take by force, and are baffled in their efforts. Regarding the body only with the purblind eyes of the anatomist, the physiologist or the pathologist, they do not see the man himself at all. Nevertheless instinct tells them he is there, somewhere. They address him, talk to him, listen to him (with a stethoscope) and order him about as if they had him completely in their power and knew all about him. But the fact is they have come nowhere near him and know next to nothing about him. Pretending a skill and insight which they do not possess, they try to hide their deficiencies in true knowledge by a display of manual and instrumental dexterity which thus becomes essentially cruel and violent. It is like vivisecting a bird to learn the secret of its song.

After diagnosis comes treatment. And here, as we turn the pages of history, we are introduced into a veritable "Chamber of Horrors," from which one is fortunate to escape with his life and a whole skin, to say nothing about his internal organs, his purse and his jewelry.

In olden times when a man got sick they shut him up in a tightly closed room, smothered him beneath blankets in a bed surrounded with heavy draperies, denied him water to quench his thirst, leeched him, bled him white, poulticed and blistered him, put moxa and setons in his quivering flesh, purged him, puked him and filled him up with all kinds of fantastic compounds of deadly drugs. It was a miracle of medical art if he came through, and "a dispensation of providence" if he did not.

Later they subjected him, amongst many other methods, to the aqueous processes of the hydropathic system. They hot and cold-packed him, hot and cold-douched and sprayed him, sitz and footbathed him, flooded him within and without, fully persuaded they were cleansing him of all his impurities.

Nowadays the patient is submitted to other forms of medical assault and battery. All the batteries and resources of "modern medical science" are turned upon him. He is X-rayed, violet-rayed, infra-red rayed and solar-rayed. He is radiumized, electrified and all but electrocuted. He is chlorine gassed, poison-sprayed, malignant-germed. He is immunized, proteinized, pollenized, endocrinized, serumized, inoculated and vaccinated. He is injected, scraped, scarified, and punctured with hypodermic needles. He is baked, boiled and "roasted." He is drugged, doped and— deluded, for when all is done he is not cured, and has actually or virtually become an "addict" of one kind or another.

If these diagnosticians and doctors were as humane as the surgeons, who mercifully anesthetize their victims before operation and studiously refrain from drugging them afterward, one could feel a little more charitable toward them. But they do not. The medical patient must "take his medicine" with as much fortitude as he can summon, smile if he can, and go his way, a victim of violence and misdirected energy. Regarding disease as an entity, something material or tangible, and not as a state of imbalance, of dynamical dysfunctioning, they naturally treat it by similar means, chemically, mechanically, materially, forcibly.

The basic idea, the fundamental therapeutic principle of "Allopathy," or orthodox medicine, is force, or violence, a maximum of means, employed in opposition and resistance. Against this stands Homeopathy, the therapeutic science and art of Vital Dynamics, based upon the idea of power, properly directed and flowing gently and smoothly along the lines of least resistance, in accordance with the laws of nature; using always a minimum of means directed toward the removal of opposition and obstruction and the restoration of harmony and balance.

It may be hard to believe because of its relevancy today, but the original full-length version of this article was written in 1927!
(Used by permission)

History has shown us that not every scientific or technological advance is beneficial to the human condition. Nuclear weapon technology is one such example. In the medical field, the diagnostic skill and insight of the family doctor of yesterday has been all but lost today in the overwhelming dependence on diagnostic equipment and the long prevailing attitude that men and women are merely complex machines. Health care is still cold, impersonal, myopic, and mechanical to an extreme.

Health care has also become an extremely huge-profit, hi-tech industry in the last several decades. Many Americans not only can't afford the high cost of health care, but are also disenchanted with the care and benefit they receive for their hard-earned dollars. The shift toward complementary and alternative health care by the general population is a positive and necessary step toward an admirable goal of achieving a well-balanced, *integrated,* and affordable health care system that works for everyone. A more humanitarian and complete system of health care is necessary, and the seeds have already begun to take root.

II

FOR EVERY WOMAN

DEALING WITH EMOTIONAL CRISES

Happiness is not the absence of conflict, but the ability to cope with it.
Author Unknown

How do we as women handle the emotional crises that befall or confront us?

I have a friend whose husband just left her, without warning, and no marital problems that she was aware of. They are both in their late thirties. They have several school-age children. Her husband simply called her up one late afternoon and told her that he'd rented an apartment and wasn't coming home.

I know another woman whose husband left her for a younger woman after 20 years of marriage. The anger she felt toward her husband consumed her thoughts for well over a year after the final divorce decree.

Another woman I know, age forty, suffers from severe arthritis. It cropped up out of seemingly nowhere nine months ago and she has been taking chemotherapy drugs just to stay mobile.

I knew another woman who wanted very badly to have a child. She found out she was infertile and for five years tried every infertility procedure known to medical science to become pregnant, to no avail.

A former coworker of mine faced the rapid deterioration and death of her 38 year-old husband from brain cancer in a mere three-month period of time.

I've known women whose young children have died. The emotional shock and sadness is devastating.

There are numerous mothers with teenagers who have drug and criminal behavior problems, and they don't know how to reach their children or alleviate the stress it's created in their lives.

A preponderance of women under the age of 40 in America are currently in a state of premature menopause, and wondering if they are going crazy because of the dramatic physical and emotional turbulence that can occur during this time in a woman's life.

Most of us will face an emotional crisis at one or more times in our lives. It doesn't mean we've done anything to deserve it, and it doesn't mean the end of the world. It does mean, however, that we all need to be armed with the ability to get through the crises we're confronted with.

There are several important things I have learned, strategies I have adopted to help me get through tough times and emotional crises. I discuss some of them here on the off chance they might be of help to someone else facing a crisis.

1. Let your emotions out, don't bottle them up. Negative emotions are poison to the human system if not released. Find a constructive way to release the grief, fear, anguish, and anger that comes with a crisis.

2. Everything comes to pass, not to stay forever. Know that time truly can and does heal emotional upheaval and that nothing stays the same indefinitely. It takes everyone time to get through the shocks, losses, setbacks, and emotional traumas of life. So give yourself the opportunity to release the emotion that comes with a crisis but likewise don't allow yourself to remain in a state of fear, sorrow, depression, or anger indefinitely. We all need to move in a forward motion with time.

3. *Don't isolate yourself from others!* Work on building an emotional support system of people in your life if you don't already have one. It can consist of family members, friends, coworkers, support group members, members of your church congregation, clergy, etc.

We all should have someone to lean on when the going gets rough, and someone to sympathize and empathize with what we're going through. Share your burdens and sorrow with others. Don't absorb it alone!

4. Have faith in a higher power and your own inner strength. The strength of both is truly amazing.

5. Don't beat yourself up about things that are out of your control. I see a lot of useless and self-defeating anger and guilt in women whose husbands have left them and mothers whose children have become substance-addicted or dropouts. We can't control the behavior and decisions of others. We can only set positive examples and implement constructive guidance when the opportunity presents itself.

6. Stay busy. Have work, hobbies, and activities to keep you occupied, so that you're not solely focused on the storm that's blown into your life. The more free time you have to dwell on a crisis situation, the bigger it can and will become in your mind. Don't have all your eggs in one basket.

7. Avoid negative people, negative television programming, negative reading material, etc. When life presents you with an emotional crisis, you don't need to add fuel to the already stressful situation by absorbing negative input and influences. Allow yourself to absorb only that which is positive.

8. Count your blessings. I never felt inclined to do this when emotionally distraught, but found that writing a list on paper of the good things and people in your life can help, especially when you've temporarily lost your perspective on life in general or the present circumstances.

9. Get involved or stay involved in helping others. Volunteer for a charity, school, or other organization with a positive worthwhile goal of helping others. This always brings positive emotional benefit to you.

10. Read, and keep readily available, positive, inspirational, and humorous reading material to provide you with an emotional lift in your day whenever you may need or want it. (I list some of my own favorite positive inspirational reading material at the end of this section simply for an example.) Since humor is more specifically a matter of personal taste, I didn't include an example listing here.

All of these things have helped me to get through each crisis situation I've faced thus far in my life, and equally important, allowed me to get past or "out of" my own feelings and emotions throughout the crisis. With time, a new and possibly empowering perspective on every ordeal can surface.

{One final note: If you or any member of your family is in a life-threatening crisis situation, seek immediate help and intervention.}

Some of my favorite inspirational reading includes the following:

TIMELESS WISDOM, A Life-Changing Quotation Book
Compiled by Gary W. Fenchuk
(Copyright 1994 by Cake Eaters, Inc.)

THE INSPIRATIONAL WRITINGS OF ROBERT H. SCHULLER:
Tough Times Never Last But Tough People Do,
and my personal favorite,
Tough Minded Faith for Tender Hearted People
(Published by Inspirational press, a division of BBS Publishing Corp.)

All the CHICKEN SOUP books including:
CHICKEN SOUP FOR THE WOMAN'S SOUL, and
CHICKEN SOUP FOR THE MOTHER'S SOUL

By Jack Canfield…et al.
(Published by Health Communications, Inc.)

THE POWER OF POSITIVE THINKING, and
TREASURY OF JOY AND ENTHUSIASM
By Norman Vincent Peale
Published by Ballantine Books.

No matter what your religion or personal spiritual philosophy, there is wonderful, inspirational literature available to you. If you don't have any positive reading material in your home at this time, please visit your local library or your favorite neighborhood bookstore. A daily dose of positive inspiration and humor can not only give you an emotional boost when you desperately need it, but can also brighten up all those days you aren't facing a crisis.

SPIRITUALITY AND RELIGION

The happiness of your life depends upon the quality of your thoughts.
Marcus Antonius

What we think, we become.
Buddha

Spirituality is individual as it comes from within.

I think most of us believe in a supremely benevolent and intelligent universal spirit, whether we choose to name it or not. I know that many individuals who develop a powerful faith in this ultimate positive power find inner strength and peace through their voluntary connection with it.

Many American women have a difficult time relating to the patriarchal image of God written and spoken of throughout the ages by men. Only by taking into account the historically egoistic and animalistic nature of men does it become possible to understand the necessity of a patriarchal God image for men (and some women). Realizing that the majority of the world's people also would have difficulty grasping the concept of a supreme universal spirit, without relating it to an image created within the limited realms of human comprehension and imagination, allows us to understand the many cultural interpretations of God presented to us throughout religious history.

I grew up with no particular religious foundation or education so found it illuminating to explore the many facets of different religions and spiritual philosophies without any predetermined influence or religious "training". Most of my friends throughout childhood and early adulthood were of Roman Catholic, Protestant, or Jewish faith. Over the years I have also met and known individuals of Oriental and Middle Eastern religions, occultists, humanists, naturalists, and individuals belonging to some of the more radical Evangelical movements that were formed in America during the 1800's.

Though I have never learned to respect beliefs that blatantly or subtly promote selective superiority, crippling superstition, hate, fear, or indifference to others, I have found some positive values in most practiced religions and spiritual philosophies. I have also discovered, however, that there are many people who have prevented themselves from developing their own character, who have avoided making any effort to improve their own circumstances or the human condition in general, who have committed all manner of "sin" and atrocities, and have quietly or vigorously condemned anyone who didn't hold their own particular beliefs—all in the name of God. What I observe in the foregoing is not "God's will", but the results of man's will and/or man's self-serving interpretation of God's will.

No religion thus far has "vaccinated" everyone against diseases of the moral character.

Life here on earth is a series of learning and growing experiences. Few if any of us are capable of abandoning self-interest entirely or of attaining a state of spiritual perfection. But, each time we reject and overcome negative, stifling, prejudicial, and destructive impulses, habits and influences, we positively progress our own character and the spiritual condition of humankind.

Whether or not we believe in an afterlife, there is no denying that we are all living lives filled with immediate and future consequences. As we invest ourselves in positive or negative living, attitudes, and beliefs here on earth, so will be the return on our investment.

I don't attempt to define or interpret God because I know my efforts would be humanly and individually flawed. Instead, I simply hold the steadfast belief that a positive, intelligent, and infinite power indeed exists, and that deep within each of us lies the wondrous ability to "plug into it".

"The Change of Life"

God grant me the serenity to accept the things I cannot change, courage
to change the things I can, and wisdom to know the difference.
Reinhold Niebuhr (Serenity Prayer)

I have read that in some countries the symptoms of PMS and menopause are not experienced or even heard of. Some logical explanations for the prevalence of these symptoms in American and Western European women are discussed in several superb books which I feel privileged to have read, and list at the end of this section for informational purposes. Our society's attitude toward menstruation, childbirth, and menopause, for the most part, is backward, chauvinistic, and unhealthy. Women can educate themselves and others in the natural wonder of these previously "taboo" topics and in so doing, improve and/or change the prevailing negative attitudes of our society.

The medical community, in its efforts to alleviate PMS and menopausal symptoms in multitudes of women, has often unintentionally created more problems for them, through the performance of many unnecessary hysterectomies and the administration of synthetic hormones with potentially dangerous side effects. For the medical community to view a woman's natural biological processes as a "handicap" is unscientific and psychologically damaging, which may explain why a growing number of women in this country are treating their own PMS and menopausal symptoms with herbs, natural progesterone cream and/or natural estrogen, homeopathy, flower essence therapy, oriental medicine, and nutritional therapy.

The symptoms of menopause can begin quite early in some women, long before the cessation of the menses. I, myself, began having hot flushes, fluid retention, dry and intensely itchy skin, and several other problematic symptoms associated with menopause at the age of 32. The majority of people in and out of the medical profession will vehemently proclaim that if you are under the age of 40, you are too young to experience any symptoms of hormonal imbalance. Let them proclaim what they will, but take the time to educate yourself on this subject.

Emotional support may be found in talking with others who are experiencing similar symptoms. If you don't know anyone personally that you feel comfortable discussing this with, there are early-menopause and menopause support groups on the Worldwide Web that can offer you an understanding ear. Always use discrimination when communicating with anyone via the computer, and remember that any helpful suggestions you may receive from laypersons are never to be used as a substitute for qualified medical help.

The following books proved helpful to me in understanding the many complexities of so-called "female problems", and also provide information on alternative and/or complementary treatment options and resources:

WHAT YOUR DOCTOR MAY *NOT* TELL YOU ABOUT
MENOPAUSE
The Breakthrough Book on Natural Progesterone
JOHN R. LEE, M.D.
With Virginia Hopkins
(Warner Books)

****

WOMEN'S BODIES WOMEN'S WISDOM
Creating Physical and Emotional Health and Healing
CHRISTIANE NORTHRUP, M.D.
(Bantam Trade Paperbacks)

****

THE PREMATURE MENOPAUSE BOOK
When the "Change of Life" Comes Too Early
KATHRYN PETRAS
(Whole Care Trade Paperbacks)

****

HORMONE REPLACEMENT THERAPY
YES OR NO?
How to Make an Informed Decision about Estrogen, Progesterone, &
Other Strategies for Dealing with PMS, Menopause and Osteoporosis
BETTY KAMEN, Ph.D.
(Nutrition Encounter)

****

Get to know your body and your self. Appreciate and enjoy all the stages of your life. They all have something wonderful to offer us, including menopause!

LIFELONG PERSONAL GROWTH

The life which is unexamined is not worth living.
Plato

Regret for the things we did can be tempered with time; it is regret
for the things we did not do that is inconsolable.
Sidney J. Harris

The topic of personal growth is hardly new, and it can mean something different to everyone. The term "midlife crisis" has had a tremendous amount of publicity in the past. I see it as a time when the long-ignored need for continued personal growth surfaces. I dislike the term midlife crisis simply because the word crisis denotes a negative event rather than a positive one. Following are two glaring examples of the negative connotations associated with the term "midlife crisis":

1. A man in mid-life leaves his wife to pursue a relationship with another (usually younger) woman, buys a sporty car, and joins a gym for the first time in his life.

2. A woman in mid-life seeks cosmetic surgery, shops for her clothes in the juniors section of a department store, and begins to frequent nightclubs trendy to the younger set.

In both cases, the futile and often disillusioning attempt to recapture youth or a bygone era in life only prevents personal growth and self-acceptance.

Many people, including myself, believe so-called "midlife crisis" would be better interpreted as a time when the stifled or ignored need for personal growth surfaces, a time when the opportunity for growth finally presents itself after years of being overridden by the responsibilities of everyday life.

So many of us spend decades (or even lifetimes) focusing all of our time and energy on making a living, taking care of our families, running errands and doing domestic chores, that we sacrifice our need for creative, educational, recreational, and spiritual pursuits. How many women might there be in America right now who are desperate for simply one day or even one hour of peace and quiet, rest and relaxation, or fun? Most of us are so overwhelmed by family and/or job responsibility that we scarcely have time to take care of ourselves, let alone pursue any personal goals.

What's the answer? Making time for our selves. Easier said than done if you've always put others before yourself, but it is possible. Some quiet time for thinking is necessary to determine in what areas of your life some responsibility could be shared by others, freeing up some of your time for personal pursuits. Spouses and older children (if you have them) can assume some of the chores and responsibilities that you may have always taken care of in the past. Grandparents, relatives, and friends are also usually willing to offer assistance to you periodically.

If you are financially able to do so, working part time instead of full time can open up a wealth of opportunity for you to pursue your own interests.

Simplifying your life and organizing your time can help, especially if you are living beyond your means or running yourself ragged doing mundane chores.

I can only offer the following meager suggestions for making time available. The actual logistics will need to be worked out on an individual basis.

If your weekends are tied up with household chores and errands, make an effort to get done what you can during the week. For example, do grocery shopping on a weekday evening, keep up with the laundry during the week so it doesn't become an all day project for Saturday, and assign daily housecleaning chores to older children if you have them.

If you don't have children old enough to help, and you can afford it, pay an outside service to clean your home regularly for you. You may have to eliminate an existing luxury from your monthly budget to afford it, but it could be well worth it. For too many of us, weekends have become more tiring and stressful than weekdays, in our harried efforts to accomplish all the chores we've neglected during the week.

If you're a single parent (which I was for four years with my first child), you really must make the most of children's naptimes, sleepovers, etc. And I don't mean that you should fill up that time paying bills or cleaning out the refrigerator. Use those welcome breaks from responsibility to do something you enjoy or to relax. Take a long bath, read something mood lifting, give yourself a pedicure, enjoy a hobby, or just meditate. It doesn't matter what you do, as long as you do it for *yourself*. Also, try to create a support network of people if you don't already have one. Family and friends can be godsends to the single parent (or anyone for that matter!), providing emotional support and reliable babysitting options which allow you time to pursue your own interests or simply get a break from your daily responsibilities.

The opposite of growth is stagnation, and we must avoid stagnation if we are to feel good about our selves and life in general. Learning new things keeps life interesting and challenges us in new and different ways. In the past year, for example, I read several books on subjects new and interesting to me; took Tai Chi, CPR, and first aid classes; taught myself tole painting and displayed my wares at a local craft show; volunteered for five months at a local elementary school; learned a new computer program; and undertook writing this book. It's amazing what can be done with a minimal amount of free time. When I take a class, it's either for one hour, one evening per week, or a one-time evening class that lasts for several hours. I volunteered during part of my youngest child's preschool hours, and did the tole painting during many of her naptimes. I often do my reading and journal writing when everyone else at home has gone to bed for the night. And during those wonderful periods when everyone at home is occupied with something (no matter for how long), I've worked on the book when not too tired to concentrate. If I don't have the energy to do anything, I do nothing. (Which I realized only recently was okay to do!) I also realized, just in the last year, that I can't accommodate everyone else's needs and ignore my own, or my nervous system gets the better of me and I end up unable to do much of anything! Being a mother of two who works part time, I do have more available free time than those parents who work full time, but when I do go back to working full time again, I will nevertheless still make time to pursue my own interests, for the sake of my sanity and well-being.

Once you've arranged some free time for yourself, you've won half the battle in fulfilling your personal growth needs.

Next, of course, is deciding what to do with the time. Anything positive you do that enriches you mentally, emotionally, or spiritually, will cause you to grow as an individual. Expand your horizons! The choices are limitless and yours to make.

III

HELPING OUR CHILDREN MAKE
POSITIVE CHOICES

INTRODUCTION

Resolve to be tender with the young, compassionate with the aged,
sympathetic with the striving, and tolerant with the weak and the
wrong. Sometime in life you will have been all of these.
Lloyd Shearer

If you can dream it, you can do it.
Walt Disney

Some parents don't discuss important issues that kids need knowledge of when entering the real world as productive adults. In general, we teach them what they need to know and do in order to be safe and healthy, and impress upon their minds our individual beliefs and value systems and the values of our society (positive or negative). Much important and practical information is not addressed or provided by parents or the public or private education systems. The following are some important topics both we, and our children need to be educated on in order to make positive life choices for ourselves:

1. Marriage
2. Parenting
3. Self-esteem.
4. Personal finance.
5. Our connection and responsibility to our Earth and nature.
6. Materialism and superficiality.

Most young children I've had the pleasure of knowing have the following idea about life: You go to school, you get a job, get married, raise children, then retire and play golf and spoil your grandchildren. Then your body wears out and dies. Many children know little or nothing about how to make positive life choices for themselves utilizing their own internal guidance systems. I believe many adults don't either.

Children gain knowledge and coping and decision-making skills through the example of others, life experience, formal education, making mistakes (learning cause and effect) and discovery (sudden insight). They learn behavior by example: the images, ideas, and people they are surrounded with or exposed to. The wisdom of the ages tells us that for them to live a positive, fulfilling and productive life, positive examples must be set for our children by all adults. To allow the creation or continuance of a society of illiterate, unethical, immoral, self-serving people only serves to insure the decay of our humanity and promote mediocrity in our quality of life.

MARRIAGE

*Be not angry that you cannot make others as you wish them to be
since you cannot make yourself as you wish to be.*
Thomas a' Kempis

I admit it. I have made some really poor choices for myself regarding relationships with men. I always naively assumed that everyone was genuinely caring, sincere, intelligent, and secure, even if that wasn't my first impression. It took me almost 15 adult years to realize that the level of maturity and positive qualities I found in a man the first few weeks of knowing him was usually about 95% of the sum total he possessed. More than once I spent over five years in an energy-draining relationship, waiting to see the qualities I was looking for, sure it was only a matter of time before they surfaced, only to finally realize I was totally mistaken. I'm not speaking of unrealistic visions of perfection, which some people seem to entertain. I was simply looking for a friend; someone I genuinely liked and respected, who shared similar values and could relate to me on more than a physical level; a positive and supportive person who wanted to mature, love, experience life, and grow together with me through the years. Which leads me to a book recommendation. If I had the opportunity to read this book as a teenager or young adult, I still may not have known what I really wanted in a mate, but I sure would have been better able to recognize what I didn't want! The book I'm referring to was written by Dr. Laura Schlessinger, the host of her own internationally syndicated radio program, author of a nationally syndicated newspaper column, and a licensed marriage, family and child counselor in the State of California. The title of the book is:

45

"*Ten Stupid Things Men Do To Mess Up Their Lives*". This wonderful book outlines the 10 major "stupid behaviors" of men. In all fairness, I must also mention that we women are not immune to "stupid behavior" patterns, and Dr. Schlessinger has written a book about us too: "*Ten Stupid Things Women Do To Mess Up Their Lives*". It's definitely beneficial to read both books, just to be sure you aren't being your own worst enemy in the realm of male/female relationships.

The person you choose to marry. Possibly 90% of the happiness or misery during your adult life will be based on this decision. If there is only one time in your life that you act rationally and intelligently without impulse or superficiality, let it be in this monumental decision!

It's probable that the younger you are, the less surety you will have about what you want in a life partner and co-parent for your children. And if you've had less than positive role models in your life, you may consciously or unconsciously attract those of the opposite sex with the same negative characteristics you grew up thinking were standard or normal. This can make things confusing, especially when physical attraction sends your hormones and emotions reeling!

Before committing to any permanent relationship, allow yourself ample time to really get to know the other person. Sure, they may look great, have a decent job, be a great dancer, drive a nice car, or practice the same religion as you, but only time can show you the real character of a person. As with any important undertaking, we need to strive to see things as they really are. The honeymoon atmosphere may not last forever, but love can.

Time is a wonderful thing. Allowing a bare minimum of a year to get to know someone is a wise decision. Give yourself a true chance to see all facets of the other's personality under a variety of conditions. Time will show you a person's temperament, emotional maturity, goals, interests; how they relate to other people in general and the quality of their family relationships and friendships; likes and dislikes, personal habits, etc. Many negative behaviors and characteristics can be uncovered with time, sparing you from making a disastrous decision. You could discover that your prospective mate spends all his free time watching television or sleeping, that he's a compulsive slob or neat-freak, that he spends money like it grows on trees or is an extreme tightwad. You could also discover more serious characteristics and behaviors, such as violent tendencies, questionable morals, emotional problems and immaturity, addictions, etc.

You need to be comfortable and compatible with the personality of the person you choose to marry. Communication with him should come easily, and it is imperative that you like and respect him the way he is. Take the time to delve beneath the surface. And before making a commitment, it's not a bad idea to seek premarital counseling or input from an objective third party if there's a chance you are blinded by the feeling of being in love. Even if you aren't, it's not a bad idea. Many churches offer pastoral counseling and compatibility testing. Regardless of whether or not you utilize any type of premarital counseling service, talk to your prospective mate in depth before marriage. Find out his views and goals regarding marriage, careers, having and raising children, domestic and parental chores, home ownership, pets, vacation time and celebration of holidays, etc. Differences need to be ironed out before marriage, not after. Know that an informed and well-thought-out decision is always easier to live with.

Ask yourself why you want to get married and make a list of your honest answers. Then review your answers to determine whether your motivations are superficial or negative. If your answers prove to be positive, then you can be confident in your decision. Here are just a few reasons people get married that could invite unhappiness and/or divorce:

1. To "trap" someone you've allowed yourself to become unhealthily dependent on. (Purposely getting pregnant without the partner's consent is a good example of "entrapment".)
2. To escape your present environment, or because of dissatisfaction with your life at present.

3.   You are marrying to spite someone else. (Such as your parents or a former love interest.)

4.   Blinded by the feeling of being in love, you haven't given yourself a chance to really know the other person.

5.   You feel pressured by family members.

6.   You feel pressured by your "biological clock" ticking away.

7.   You are marrying for personal gain, whether financial, social, career, etc.

8.   You don't have a permanent mindset in regard to marriage. Divorce is always an option in your mind if things don't work out the way you wanted them to.

9.   To "rescue" someone from himself or his current situation, believing your love will transform him.

10. You're bored.

11. Feeling unloved and insecure, you're latching onto the first person that shows you some attention and affection.

12. You see the opportunity to dominate another person or be dominated yourself.

13. Fear of living independently, because you lack the drive or confidence to make a life for yourself.

If you recognize any of these reasons as your own, don't get married yet. Wait until you can marry for positive reasons. On the other hand, if your motives have proven themselves to be positive and you've given yourself enough time to know the true character of your intended (and you still love him!) then congratulations are in order! You're embarking on a wonderful and rewarding partnership.

PARENTING

When a man dies, if he can pass enthusiasm along to his children,
he has left them an estate of incalculable value.
Thomas Edison

Having and raising children is not an easy task. The rewards can be magnificently wonderful, and the trials equally harrowing. Children require among other things, love, nurturing and support, positive role models, and emotional security. Be sure that your motivations for having and raising children are positive, and not negative or self-serving.

I've known teenagers who purposely became pregnant in an attempt to try to hold onto a boyfriend, or to get out of their parents home, or because they wanted someone to love them and thought a child was the answer. (Without realizing the tremendous responsibility they were undertaking.)

I've known adults who had children in order to receive larger public assistance checks, or in hopes the child would hold a failing relationship together.

I've known people with abusive partners, or abusive themselves, who had children, knowing full well that the child or children would be subject to physical, mental, emotional, or sexual abuse. A persons or couple's motivation for wanting children must be positive and responsible, or the consequences will be negative for both parent and child. If you cannot provide a positive, safe, healthy, and loving environment for a child to grow up in, *please* delay parenting until you can.

On the flip side, I have also known some wonderful parents and role models for children, and couples who longed for a child and couldn't conceive so unselfishly adopted. I salute and congratulate all positive, responsible, and loving parents and role models. Children are the future!

Having been a child myself and being a parent now, I of course have my own ideas about parenting. Like everyone else, I don't know all the answers; I never had a manual to refer to, but do the best I can and learn as I go. There are different parenting styles, and one is not necessarily better than another.

Here are a few measly parenting tidbits I've learned through my own experience and the experience of friends or family members. Some may be humorous, others serious.

1. Don't jiggle or bounce a baby after drinking milk. Chances are you'll be spit up on.
2. Don't overfeed a baby or overheat their milk. You'll be spit up on.
3. Don't lay babies on their stomach in the crib. One of my daughters would actually smash her face into the crib mattress and hyperventilate to the point of passing out! When she was old enough to turn her head and body over by herself she didn't do it any more. I never figured out why she did it in the first place, but once I was aware of the problem I lied her down on her back at all times to be safe.
4. If you've never changed a boy baby's diaper, guard yourself against getting "sprayed" mid-change!
5. Babies and toddlers seem to eat what they need. No need to worry if they go through a fruit, oatmeal, or strained yams only period. You can always supplement the baby food diet with liquid vitamins if it makes you feel better and you have your pediatrician's okay.
6. It's allright to cry when your toddler takes his/her first steps.

7. Don't take kids to the doctor every time their nose runs. If it's minor, allow their immune system do its job, so they'll be better able to stave off the next virus that comes around. And remember that antibiotics don't work on viral infections.

8. Cow's milk, sugar, and wheat are a few of the common food sensitivities that can cause children problems. If your child gets chronic ear or respiratory infections, rashes, or stomachaches, be a diet detective. If they seem to be "wired" most of the time, eliminate the candy, cookies, chocolate, and sugary or artificially sweetened drinks and processed foods from their diet. Practice eating healthful foods.

9. Set rules of conduct and behavior and provide appropriate consequences for breaking them. Be consistent.

10. Be genuinely interested in what they say and do.

11. Know their friends. Know the home environment of their friends.

12. Set a positive example!

13. Help them discover talents and find hobbies and activities they will enjoy, and encourage them to be productive and involved. Teach them to be resourceful. There's nothing worse than the unending whine of: "I'm bored, there's nothing to do!"

14. Give children responsibilities as soon as they are old enough to assume them. It will teach them to give of themselves unselfishly and also to be a productive member of the family unit. The positive habits of cleaning up after themselves, keeping their own room neat, and helping out other family members when needed should be learned early on.

15. Don't allow an allowance or reward to become their sole motivation for accomplishing tasks or helping others.

16. Help them with and check their homework. Attend their school plays, band concerts, and athletic events. Join the PTA. Go to Open House night. Be involved in their lives and education.

17. Relay to older children the vital connection between education and their future job prospects.
18. Don't buy them everything they want. If you do they may not learn to appreciate what they do have (counting their blessings), live within their means, or enjoy the simple things in life.
19. Don't be surprised or hurt if at some point in their life your child tells you that you don't understand him or her. It usually means that they don't understand themselves.
20. Don't ignore your kids or allow them to do whatever they want. They need structure, supervision, and consequences to negative behavior to feel secure.
21. Fear, worry, hate, envy, and prejudice are learned, not born into us. Teach your children to challenge themselves more than others, especially male children who have traditionally been encouraged mostly to compete against others.
22. Love, teach, and inspire your children.

The Preteen and Teen Years

I've made a separate subsection for this period in the lives of parents and children because it can be an exasperating time. I have been through some *very* stressful times with my teenager, so I speak from experience.

Hormonal changes occur during this time, and emotional changes along with them. This transitional period between wanting to remain a child and wanting to become an adult is usually not easy. Many times children rebel against their parents and the "status quo" in their quest for independence and individuality. Since we can't be with them every minute, there are times when we have to trust them to make their own decisions and do the right thing.

Peer pressure is prevalent during this time, and no matter how responsible, caring, and supportive a parent you have been, certain personalities may be inclined to experiment or participate in negative or self-destructive behavior. How can you prevent it from happening? There's no guaranteed method of prevention short of shipping them off to military school, but if the family foundation is solid and positive, you're one step ahead of the game.

I have learned the hard way that any free time an adolescent has will be filled one way or another. Encourage and promote hobbies, music and dance, athletics, club and/or church activities, etc. so your child doesn't fill his or her time up with self-destructive pursuits and people. It's a lot easier to get into trouble when you have a lot of free time on your hands. Encourage involvement in worthwhile activities and causes while kids are in elementary school and it will most likely carry over into middle school, high school, and adulthood. Kids need to be busy doing things they enjoy and that help them grow as human beings. Adults do, too!

If your child becomes chronically involved in negative or self-destructive activities, your heart-to-heart talks are falling on deaf ears, your disciplinary measures have proven ineffective and the behavior is creating a stressful environment for other family members, don't be embarrassed or hesitate to seek help from a family counselor, pastor, or other appropriate outside service. Sometimes an objective third party can help to solve the problem. If you've reached that point where you've exhausted every available resource and option in an attempt to remedy the situation and nothing has worked, you may have to let it go and simply pray for all parties involved. This may sound corny to some of you, but prayer is a powerful tool if you're willing to use it, and it's not just for use in emergency situations. Faith and prayer can be of comfort and may help hold together what seems to be falling apart. You don't have to belong to a church to have faith and pray. You need only to believe in a universal positive power greater than yourself and your problems, that which we call God.

Positive Ideas and Rules for Children:

1. The amount of benefit we receive from years of formal education and self-education is a direct result of how much effort and enthusiasm we put into learning.

2. Live and love by the Golden Rule: "Do unto others as you would have them do unto you." I like to expand on this by including: Say nothing to or about others that you would not want people saying to or about you. Treat people as you expect to be treated, with respect and kindness.

3. Choose your friends wisely. Negative influences, thoughts, and actions produce negative results. Associate with positive, productive people, be positive and productive yourself, and you can expect positive results.

4. Don't put all your eggs (or energy) in one basket. This applies to friends and associates, interests, aspirations, all areas of life where limits will restrict your personal growth.

5. Believe in yourself, your inner strength and ability. Know that you can rise above any difficulty with determination and positive faith.

6. Continually set new goals for yourself throughout life. Always have something to work toward and look forward to. Doing so will prevent boredom and self-destructive attitudes and behavior, build and improve self-esteem, and help you realize your self-worth.

7. Strive for balance in all areas of your life.

8. Be yourself and the best self you can be.

9. Accept responsibility for your own actions!

Self-esteem

Associate reverently, and as much as you can, with your loftiest thoughts.
Henry David Thoreau

Many of us lack confidence in ourselves, and how we feel about ourselves determines how we will relate to others, how they will relate to us, and what we will seek to achieve in our lifetimes. But, we are not born with the spirit of fear or insecurity.

How you feel about yourself by the time you reach adulthood can be largely determined by the external influences in your life up to that point. Your parent(s) or guardian(s) are your first and primary influence. To be loved, nurtured, provided with positive principals for living and relating to others, to be supported and encouraged to learn and grow in every respect, to learn to be true to yourself and respectful of others and all life; these are just a few of the important, positive things we need to learn and receive from our parents/guardians growing up. For parents to set negative examples of destructive or violent/abusive behavior, indifference, or neglect is to create disastrous consequences for both child and parent. The "dysfunctional family" is all too prevalent in our society. Destructive cycles of behavior have to stop entirely if we are to view and live life as a gift to be enjoyed and not a problem to be solved. Friends can have tremendous influence over us, as well, especially during the adolescent years when the search for our individuality and independence becomes a driving internal force. A favorite greeting card I bought read: "Friends are the family we choose for ourselves." This is true, so we must therefore make wise choices in this area throughout our lives.

All the people we don't know personally, especially all those involved in media advertising and entertainment, also have tremendous potential to influence our character and values.

If you've been blessed with a positive support system (family, friends, teachers, etc.) growing up, you probably won't have a deficiency of self-confidence when you reach adulthood. However, if the people closest to you have imprinted you with negative information and experiences throughout your childhood, you will probably need to acknowledge and share these negatives with a positive, caring person who has perhaps over-come similar influences and experiences, to attain a perspective on life that will be a positive healing force for you. Tragedy can turn into triumph when the tragedy teaches others the consequences of negative actions and/or provides them with viable preventative information and strategies.

Though we cannot choose our parents when we're born, nor our imme-diate and extended family members, we can choose all the other people we invite into our lives. And in choosing, we must remember that negative is not the norm, even if our environment or support system of people grow-ing up was negative. (That's why all the news is so dismal it's the negative stories and events that make headlines because positive is the usual state of affairs.)

We can increase our sense of self-worth by *letting go* of the past negative influences and experiences impressed upon us by others over whom we had no control over. We must remember that the only spirit we can con-trol is our own, and it is imperative that we make positive choices for our-selves. Make well thought out, positive, and fulfilling choices throughout your life, and remain ever true to yourself. Seek out and find people who will fill you instead of drain you. Those who encourage and support you, instead of discourage you or diminish your enthusiasm, and people who instill hope and courage in you, instead of cynicism and fear. Those who will love and respect you, not use, abuse, or stifle you. Those who accept you just as you are and don't discriminate against you out of ignorance or their own self-righteousness. It's also important to remember to be your own best friend.

Most people are basically well meaning, and good-hearted. Learning to recognize and discern the good from the bad in people is easy for some people, but for those who have open and trusting personalities by nature it can be quite a trick. To do so may require input from *objective* people if you haven't quite got the knack for it yet. Once you let go of the past and forgive yourself for mistakes, allow your internal guidance and warning system and your own wisdom and knowledge lead you into a confident and positive future.

PERSONAL FINANCE

A fool and his money soon part.
English Proverb

All of us have to learn the basics about money somewhere, and home is the logical place. When children are young, teach them the value of each coin and a dollar bill. Relate the value of the money to things they could purchase such as a coloring book or a toy. I took my four-year-old to the store with a dollar to show her what she could buy with it and what she couldn't. She learned that she could buy Barbie stickers with the dollar, but not a Barbie doll. She now understands (no matter how abstractly) that sometimes you have to save up your coins and dollars to buy something you don't have enough money for now.

When kids are in elementary school or junior high, you can show them the realities of paychecks and monthly bills. Have children sit with you through a bill-paying session when they are old enough to understand the concepts of money and bills, and they will learn that house payments, groceries, utilities, and medical bills have to be paid first before new clothes, a new toy, or going to the movies can even be considered.

If they are given an allowance, teach them to save at least a portion of it for a future major expense such as a car when they are of legal age to drive. The sense of accomplishment they would feel when you actually took them car-shopping with the money they'd saved would be priceless.

When kids are old enough to legally work, encourage them to get a part-time job, but not one with so many hours that their schoolwork suffers. Cut off their allowance at that point or agree to put the allowance amount in an interest bearing account for them as long as they work and save a specified portion of their pay. With your contribution, and the earned interest on their bank account, you'll be showing them that they can make money by saving money. Also, introduce them to savings bonds, mutual funds, and other investment options at this point. By the time your child is a teenager and old enough to work, give them an educational and helpful book on managing personal finance. I like the *Personal Finance for Dummies* book by Eric Tyson.

High school and college age children need to be armed with honest information about credit, budgeting, saving, and investing. Without such knowledge they could fall into serious debt accumulation habits or be ill equipped to manage their own money throughout adult life. A sound book or course on personal finance can be an invaluable asset to anyone.

Our Connection and Responsibility to our Earth and Nature

If we could see the miracle of a single flower clearly, our whole life would change.
Buddha

In nature there is balance. It is evident in the food chain, evident in the cycles of sunlight and darkness, the seasons, life and death, etc. Humankind tends to forget its connection to other living things and that our survival depends on the intricate and delicate balance of nature. We are extremely aware of our need for sunlight, water, food, and each other in order to survive and thrive, but need to be reminded of the following.

As our capacity for intelligence and emotion is the greatest of all species of life, our capability for upsetting or destroying the balance between the negative and positive forces within ourselves and nature is also the greatest.

As the largest population of users and manipulators of our environment, it is our responsibility to do our genuine best to maintain balance between what we receive from nature and what we give back. A simple example is trees: cutting down existing trees for lumber use and, in turn, planting new trees to give back what we took. Without *give* and take, we risk depletion of or destruction of the natural resources that we and our children and all future generations need to survive.

When we realize that the survival of our species depends upon the protection of the environment and wilderness areas that produce the plant, mineral, and animal life necessary for production of healing medicine and provide us with clean water to drink and clean air to breathe, we can realize the full impact of respecting our earth and nature.

After all, does it make more sense to have to chemically purify water sources we've polluted and suffer the possible or inherent long-term health risks of continual ingestion of these chemicals, or is it more logical to prevent the pollution in the first place?

We need to keep the consequences associated with our actions in the forefront of our minds at all times. As with all things, the old saying, "an ounce of prevention is worth a pound of cure", is pure and simple truth.

Little things can make a big difference. Recycling, refusing to litter and illegally dump, walking-biking-bussing to cut down on air pollution, planting trees where there are none, are just a trickle of things we as individuals can do as a matter of course to improve the polluted condition of the environment that we have collectively created. Business, industry, and government have the power to make positive global change whenever they are wise enough to take action. We can continue to contribute to or ignore the problem of our polluted environment, or we can actively work to solve it. The choice is ours to make.

MATERIALISM AND SUPERFICIALITY

Money is not required to buy one necessity of the soul.
Henry David Thoreau

Our society today is overwhelmed by and obsessed with the pursuit of material things and instant gratification. My brother likes a quotation he read in a quotation book at some point in his life that said: "Money may not buy happiness, but it provides a wider choice of miseries!" Money is a necessity in acquiring the basics of food, housing, and clothing. It is also required in the pursuit of higher education, which has also become a necessity in any society competing economically in a world market. Luxuries (everything except the basic necessities for survival) are secondary. In spite of this fact, the positive ideals and values of many people become disintegrated by a superficial and meaningless quest for material wealth and possessions, in order to distinguish themselves from the masses or gain approval from others.

I often ask myself where the personal benefit is in spending time, energy, and money striving to conform to someone else's ideal of beauty or success. Although I see it as healthy and beneficial to pamper yourself in a manner you can afford, I consider it detrimental to your pocketbook and psyche to focus exaggerated attention on (or accumulate debt in) the pursuit of physical perfection or things.

"You can't take it with you" is a true statement, but I feel it is equally wise to remember that the intangible qualities of love, friendship, hope, faith, and charity are by far more valuable and essential in the pursuit of happiness throughout life. I don't mean to say that it is undesirable or wrong to want money or things that make life a little easier or bring enjoyment; rather, that it is in our best interest to keep a healthy perspective in regard to our material and oftentimes superficial society.

No amount of material wealth or physical attributes will make people love, respect, or appreciate us for who we are. Acceptance of our selves and others comes from *within*, not from without. I feel it is important for us to remember that the examples we set for our children today will shape the character of our country tomorrow.

IV

THE NEW MILLENIUM

CLOSING THOUGHTS

If we do not change our daily lives, we cannot change the world.
Thich Nhat Hanh

Every man is a creature of the age in which he lives; very few are
able to raise themselves above the ideas of the time.
Voltaire

Death is not the greatest loss in life. The greatest loss is what dies
inside of us while we live.
Norman Cousins

My grandmother grew up in an America where women finally won the right to vote, but still were not expected to have an intelligent, independent thought about anything beyond domestic concerns. A high school diploma was desirable for a woman to have, but beyond that, what she really needed was a husband. Becoming *Mrs. Anybody* gave her an adult identity and an acceptable role in society.

My mother grew up during the Great Depression and World War II, when "true grit" was a way of life and heroes were plentiful. She read books, listened to radio, and frequented movie palaces where "bad words" were never heard on-screen and love scenes "faded out" to preserve the ideal of true (romantic) love. Whether or not the movie hero wore a white hat, he always stood out as the noblest or most confident *white man* in a crowd scene.

I grew up during the American ascendancy of television, where the real ongoing tragedies and ugliness of war, poverty, and racial and gender injustice were seen and heard nightly in the living room (between blaring commercial messages and nothing-like-life sitcoms). Girls as well as boys went off to large crowded colleges where they could not only pursue degrees but also ride the tidal waves of social protest movements. This was the postwar generation that was too massive, too visible, and too audible to be tempered by pretense or moderation.

My children are growing up in the advanced technology age of America, where instant access, instant gratification, and artificial/virtual everything is blurring (and in some cases, possibly erasing) the very humanity that makes us more precious than anything our scientific and technological zeal can produce.

The world changes so rapidly now that we can't assimilate everything our children are falling heir to, let alone evaluate it fully. Too often and in too many areas of life, we are allowing other people to think and make choices for us.

We may wish we could travel back in time to a simpler life or leap ahead into a more perfect future world, but we can't. We are where we are today because we cause our world to run like a great grandfather clock, the pendulum ever swinging back and forth from one extreme to another. At extremes, a society can't continue to thrive; that's where anarchy and tyranny are.

A senior citizen friend of mine appreciates having the time to think for herself, and comes up with some interesting ways of looking at contemporary extremism. She saw the baby-boomers anti-smoking agenda as a *feel-good* substitute for winning the war on drugs, when that battle was failing and there was no end in sight. Occasionally she sees anti-abortion demonstrations on national news, and she recognizes the participants, for the most part, as religious people on a holy crusade. But she notices that they also have chosen the easy target. She wonders why they are so obsessed with saving unborn babies when they should be able to hear the screams of all the abused and neglected babies and children who have already been born into awful circumstances.

When things have "gone too far" in our society, our tendency is to get up on our high horse, identify some perceived enemies, and arm our selves with weapons of negativity against them. Doing so, of course, is counter-productive and offers no resolution to our problems.

The excesses and abuses in America since World War II are not the result of idealizing peace, love and equality, but are the potential hazards of progressive change actualized.

The excessive self-absorption and exaggerated materialism of Americans in recent decades has perpetuated the "anything goes" society we currently own.

American men and women need to achieve balance, integrity, tolerance, and humanity in all aspects of their lives here together. Each of us must assume equal responsibility for creating and maintaining a society of positive, meaningful values.

Each generation experiences a different world from every other generation, but we are all part of the same family.

How can we make our health, our lives, and our world better in the new millenium? By utilizing positive and constructive thought, action, and example, each one of us. Not just when we feel the urge, but consistently in everything we do. And we would be wise to remember the timeless words of Aristotle:

"Happiness is found in the golden middle of two extremes."

CONCLUSION

The individual choices we make throughout our lives can provide us with the learning experiences we need to grow and evolve into fully integrated parts of this great whole called humankind.

There is something to learn from each of our individual and collective experiences, and the knowledge we acquire from these experiences can be beneficial and/or empowering to us, regardless of whether we interpret the experiences as positive or negative in essence.

I encourage any of you who are experiencing physical, mental, or emotional distress, to firstly look inside yourself, and then all around you, for the answers that will empower you to change your life into the positive and healthy expression of living creation it can and should be.

I wish all of you health and happiness.

About the Author

Bryana C. Hillman is a certified Bach Flower Practitioner and a current member of the National Center for Homeopathy in Alexandria, VA. She is currently working toward a Diploma in homeopathy through the British Institute of Homeopathy and Complementary Medicine. A mother of two, she resides in the state of Nevada.

GLOSSARY

Bach Flower Essences: 38 flower essences derived exclusively from non-poisonous plants and trees (with the exception of Rock Water, which is derived from specific sources of natural spring water). The natural healing power of these essences targets the mental/emotional level and restores balance to the whole of an individual who may or may not be displaying physical symptoms of illness. Discovered by Dr. Edward Bach (1886-1936).

Homeopathy: A system of medicine used by millions of people worldwide for over 200 years, homeopathy was developed by a German physician named Samuel Hahnemann in the late 1700's. Homeopathy is based on the principle of "like cures like" meaning if a substance can create certain symptoms in a healthy individual, then it can stimulate the immune system to heal itself in a sick person with similar symptoms. Homeopathy treats the whole person: physical, mental, and emotional. Classical homeopathy selects and utilizes one (constitutional) remedy based on the totality of an individual, including his/her symptoms, which will stimulate the immune system to heal itself, whereas homeopathy in general may make use of several different remedies at the same time in an effort to stimulate healing. Many homeopathic medicines are available over-the-counter.

Book Description

Life Doesn't Have To Make You Sick is a personal and practical guide for women who want to take control of their health and happiness.

When conventional medicine failed to solve her chronic health conditions, the author turned to alternative and complementary medicine and met with successful results.

After years of extensive self-education and self-discovery, she can now offer women insightful, common sense strategies for achieving physical and mental/emotional health.

Through such subjects as alternative health care, dealing with emotional crises, marriage, parenting, and personal growth, the author shares her own experiences and encourages women to empower themselves in every area of their life.